# Jane Brody's

# Cold and Flu Fighter

OTHER BOOKS BY JANE BRODY

*Jane Brody's Nutrition Book*

*Jane Brody's The* New York Times *Guide to Personal Health*

*Jane Brody's Good Food Book*

*Jane Brody's Good Food Gourmet*

*Jane Brody's Good Seafood Book*

# Jane Brody's
# Cold and Flu Fighter

JANE E. BRODY

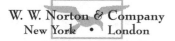
W. W. Norton & Company
New York  ·  London

The text of this book is composed in Aldine and DellaRobbia
with the display set in Bernhard Modern
This book was composed on desktop using Aldus Pagemaker 5.0
Manufacturing by The Courier Companies, Inc.
Book design and composition by Justine Burkat Trubey

**Library of Congress Cataloging-in-Publication Data**
Brody, Jane E.
[Cold and flu fighter]
Jane Brody's cold and flu fighter / by Jane E. Brody.
  p.    cm.
1. Cold (Disease)—Popular works. 2. Influenza—Popular works.
I. Title.
RF361.B76 1996
616.2'05—dc20                                        95-10236

ISBN 0-393-03913-7
ISBN 0-393-31353-0 (pbk.)

W. W. Norton & Company, Inc., 500 Fifth Avenue, New York, N.Y. 10110

W. W. Norton & Company Ltd., 10 Coptic Street, London WC1A 1PU

1  2  3  4  5  6  7  8  9  0

# CONTENTS

# Jane Brody's

# Cold and Flu Fighter

# INTRODUCTION

Y ou certainly know how you feel—*BAD*: achy, tired, with a stuffed
head, a tickle in your chest, and a throat that might have been rubbed
down with sand paper. But do you know what you have? Is it **the
flu**, debilitating and, for some, potentially deadly? Or is your at-
tacker one of the more than 200 varieties of viruses that can cause
the pesky but rarely dangerous **common cold**?

The question is not just a matter of idle medical curiosity. Knowing what you have, and what you can expect to happen to you in
the days ahead, can and should determine how you treat yourself
and those around you. Despite the difficulties people have in dis-
tinguishing a cold from the flu (a confusion aided and abetted by
the dozens of over-the-counter remedies for "colds and flu"), the
two ailments actually share little more than the fact that they are
both viral infections that attack through the respiratory system. But
the viruses responsible are light-years apart in how they behave.

1

Just as you wouldn't punish a mischievous child in the same way as you would a dishonest one, neither should you treat colds and flu as if they were one and the same.

Besieged by advice from advertisers, well-meaning friends, and enthusiasts for health foods, vitamins and other supplements, and beguiled by the nostrums of homeopathy, naturopathy, and other quasi-medical disciplines, many people end up overtreating or mistreating their symptoms. And in the process they often make matters worse. Possibly the most serious common error is to press the doctor for a prescription for antibiotics, which are useless against the viruses that cause colds and flu. When antibiotics are overused (and inappropriate use is a form of overuse), they can lose their power over the bacterial infections they are designed to treat.

Children are especially likely to receive unnecessary and sometimes harmful cold remedies ministered by over-anxious, if well-meaning, parents who feel they must do something other than watch youngsters "suffer" with the sniffles for a few days. Although children are the primary vectors of colds and frequently spread them to parents, siblings, and friends, they are also the least bothered by them, and recover from them more quickly than adults do.

# THE SHIVERY STATISTICS

At any given moment, some 30 million Americans are sneezing, coughing, blowing, shivering, or otherwise suffering through the miseries of our species' leading ailment, the common cold. In the course of a year, Americans fall victim to half a billion attacks by cold viruses. Children average six colds a year, adults one to three (more, however, if they live with young children). Even if you are now cold-free, chances are three in four that within the next year one or more of those nasty cold viruses will find you with your guard down and deliver a left hook that sends you bouncing off the ropes. Though your head may spin a bit, you'll most likely be able to get right back into the fight, cold or no cold.

The flu is another matter. It packs a punch that typically sends you to the mat. Try to get up too soon and you're likely to find yourself reeling. Luckily, few people get the flu more than once a year and most people get it only once every several years, if that often. The annual incidence of flu—or influenza, to use its proper name—varies greatly depending upon the fickleness of the virus. Most years about 10 percent of Americans—or 2.4 million people—get the flu, but in a so-called epidemic year as much as a quarter of the population may be attacked by a flu virus that manages to sneak past preexisting immunological barriers by changing its genetic footprint.

An attack by a particular flu virus leads to long-lasting immunity that enables your body to fight off subsequent attacks attempted by this same virus. There are only three basic types of flu virus—A, B, and C—but only A and B are responsible for flu epidemics. Both can undergo genetic changes that allow them to skirt around your hard-won immunity and make you as sick as you might become if you had no prior protection. When such a change occurs, especially in the more deadly type A flu virus, as many as 60 million Americans can expect to get the flu that year and more than 40,000 are likely to die from its complications. In an average year, influenza and its complications kill 10,000 to 20,000 Americans, most of whom are either elderly or already hobbled by a chronic illness like heart disease or emphysema.

Unlike colds, which can plague us year-round (the higher incidence in fall and winter is more a function of our changing behaviors than of any particular season when cold viruses flourish), flu in this country is decidedly a winter phenomenon. The flu season typically begins in November or December and peters out in March or April.

But while the flu is clearly more devastating than a cold, the very frequency of colds makes them a more costly illness. Colds are the leading medical reason for missing school or work. Each year, they account for more than 25 million lost school days and 21 million lost workdays, and that's not counting those who go to school or work with a cold but function there at less than full steam. Medically, colds eat up a significant portion of the family budget. Among children alone, colds account for more than 13 million doctor visits each year, and Americans shell out over $2.3 billion a year on medications to treat colds.

# WHAT HAVE YOU GOT?

## THE ALL-TOO-COMMON COLD

Possibly, the easiest way to tell a cold from the flu is by how your illness begins. Chances are you have a cold if the illness creeps up on you, starting perhaps with a slight sore throat or a sickly feeling beneath your ears or even a few sneezes and sniffles. The cold then gradually develops into a perpetually runny or stuffy nose, possibly accompanied by a full-fledged sore throat and hacking cough. Though you may feel slightly chilled and achy, your fever, if any, will rarely exceed 100°F (although infants and young children sometimes run fevers up to 102°F), your aches will be mild, and in most cases you'll be able to go about your usual business, albeit at a somewhat slower pace, while the cold runs its course, usually within a week to ten days.

## FLATTENED BY THE FLU

But if you are suddenly flattened as if ambushed from behind, with a high fever (102° to 104°F is common), headache, extreme fatigue and weakness, and severe aches and pains in muscles you didn't know you had, most likely you've got the flu. Upper respiratory symptoms like runny or stuffy nose and sneezing only sometimes accompany the flu. Whereas the sore throat that occurs with a cold typically disappears in a day or two, when you have the flu and your throat is sore, the soreness is likely to get worse by the second or third day. Also, the muscle aches that accompany flu are usually much more severe than you might experience with other fever-inducing ailments.

With flu, the lower respiratory tract is a common site of attack, resulting in a dry, hacking cough that can become severe. Sometimes the digestive tract also takes a beating, with vomiting and diarrhea, especially in children. When flu hits below the belt, it can be a challenge to keep down anything more nourishing than tea and water. But this symptom of influenza is not to be confused with the so-called intestinal flu, which isn't any kind of flu at all and is not accompanied by the fever, aches, pain, and severe malaise that characterizes the real flu. Because a number of infectious agents, including some bacteria, can produce flulike symptoms, people tend to use the word "flu" to describe a host of ailments that are not really influenza and are rarely as dangerous as the real thing.

Working—or playing—through the flu is usually impossible, unless you're the type who can walk on hot coals and feel no pain.

Most victims wisely (not that they have much choice) take to their beds for three or more days. The main symptoms of flu—high fever, headache, aches, and prostrating exhaustion—tend to disappear almost as suddenly as they begin, usually after three to seven days. But even after you recover, a lingering fatigue and weakness can persist for weeks and leave you with a dragged-down feeling that is sometimes compounded by depression, a common legacy of the flu virus.

## COULD IT BE AN ALLERGY?

People sometimes confuse allergies with colds. Allergies are typically seasonal, although allergies to molds, dust, and pets can occur year-round. Fever rarely accompanies an allergy attack, and while allergy symptoms can be extremely annoying and fatiguing, you're unlikely to experience that overall sick feeling that often occurs with a cold. Although the sneezing and runny nose that allergies can cause mimic the symptoms of a cold, intensely itchy eyes and nose are nearly always a sign of allergy.

Perhaps most telling is the duration: an allergic reaction to something you are only momentarily exposed to (say, someone's dog or cat) will last at most a day or two, although if the allergen is omnipresent the symptoms can persist for many weeks. A cold, on the other hand, usually lasts for seven to ten days. About one-quarter of cold victims have symptoms for two weeks or longer, and an unfortunate 10 percent are plagued for three weeks or more, even if no complications develop. Still others complain that they seem to get one cold after another, perhaps because they have temporarily exhausted their immunological defenses.

## BE WARY OF BACTERIAL INVASIONS

Sometimes, though, when a cold persists or causes debilitating pain or fever, it is no longer a cold at all but has progressed into a bacterial infection either in the sinuses (sinusitis) or middle ear (otitis media). These infections have a chance to gain a foothold when cold symptoms interfere with proper drainage in the upper respiratory passages. When a cold persists for weeks, the nasal discharge becomes thick and yellow or greenish, and a headache or painful pressure develops in the face, cheeks, upper teeth, and/or around the eyes, sinusitis is the likely cause. An ear infection is more readily recognized: the intense pain and sense of fullness in the ear is unmistakable. Only when such complicating infections arise is it time to bring in the heavy artillery—antibiotics that can attack the troublesome bacteria even though they are useless against the original viral infection.

There is no point in using antibiotics if the complicating infection is caused by a virus. Bacteria attack from outside of cells. Antibiotics used against bacteria don't work against viruses because viruses live and multiple inside cells and the antibiotics used against bacteria do not get into cells.

To add to the confusion, cold and flulike symptoms sometimes mimic more serious bacterial illnesses. Strep throat, for example, often begins like a cold, with a sore throat and fever. However, in strep throat, which is caused by a bacterium, the sore throat very quickly becomes severe, making swallowing even water problematic, fever runs high, and sometimes the heart beats rapidly. With strep throat, which should be diagnosed with a throat culture, antibiotic therapy is critically important to prevent the bacteria from causing a more serious infection of the heart valves (rheumatic fever) or the kidneys (glomerulonephritis).

## TABLE 1: IS IT A COLD OR THE FLU?

Both the common cold and influenza are upper respiratory viral infections, but the flu is a more severe and far more dangerous illness that can cause fatal complications in some people. Here's how to tell the difference.

| Symptoms | Cold | Flu |
|---|---|---|
| Onset | Gradual and mild | Sudden and severe |
| Fever | None or mild (below 100°F) | Always and high (102°– 104°F), lasting 3–4 days |
| Chills | Only if fever | Usual |
| Prostration | Rare | Prominent, early onset |
| Aches and pains | Slight | Often intense |
| Headache | Slight, if any | Prominent |
| Fatigue and weakness | Mild | Extreme, may last 2–3 weeks |
| Shortness of breath | Rare | Occasional |
| Runny or stuffy nose | Common | Occasional |
| Sneezing | Common | Occasional |
| Sore throat | Early, lasting 1–2 days | Common and often worse by 2nd or 3rd day |
| Chest discomfort, cough | If any, usually mild to moderate | Common, can become severe hacking, painful, mucus-producing cough |
| Diarrhea and vomiting | Rare | Sometimes, especially in children |

## TABLE 2: IS IT A COLD OR AN ALLERGY?

It is often hard to tell the difference between a cold and an allergy. An allergy can make a person miserable, but with a cold you are more likely to feel sick. Allergic symptoms often can be prevented by avoiding the allergen (e.g., cats for a cat allergy), by taking antihistamines, or by undergoing a lengthy series of desensitization injections (e.g., for pollen allergies).

| Characteristics | Cold | Allergy |
|---|---|---|
| Susceptibility | Anyone, any time | Usually starts in childhood or early adulthood, rarely after midlife |
| Duration | Usually 7–10 days | Usually seasonal, with specific triggers; sometimes year-round |
| Fever | Sometimes, mild | Rare |
| Aches and pains | Slight | Never |
| Itchy eyes and nose | Slight, if any | May be severe |
| Sneezing | Common | Common |
| Runny or stuffy nose | Common | Common |

# HOW DID YOU GET IT?

## COLDS ARE HARD TO CATCH

If the cold that ran through your family or your office like a hurricane, knocking down everyone in its path, has finally caught up to you, you may find this hard to believe: colds are not that easy to catch. Myths and old wives' tales notwithstanding, you do not catch colds by sitting in a draft, going out with a wet head, failing to wear a hat in winter, swimming in icy waters, getting overheated or chilled, or facing any other such environmental stress, including sudden changes in the weather.

Rather, you catch colds from other people who are already infected with a virus to which you have no preexisting immunity. Undue stress (especially the kind that results in disrupted sleep and haphazard meals), health-robbing habits like cigarette smoking and alcohol abuse, and preexisting health problems like asthma and chronic bronchitis can interfere with your body's immunological defenses and render you more susceptible to a cold. But you won't get sick unless you are also exposed to a cold virus to which you are susceptible.

Perhaps you try to keep your distance from someone with a cold. But it's not just obviously sick people who can give you their colds. Between one-half and three-fourths of those infected with cold viruses have no symptoms. In other words, they do not even know they might be capable of spreading cold viruses to other people and so are unlikely to take any special precautions. In addition, there is an incubation period of one to four days after a person becomes infected but before cold symptoms appear. During this time, the virus could unwittingly be spread to others. Any one of us, then, can be a Typhoid Mary of the common cold.

## HOW THE VIRUS GETS AROUND

Depending upon whose research you choose to believe, colds are spread from person to person in either, or both, of two ways: (1) from a hand contaminated with a cold virus to the hand (sometimes via a door knob or telephone) of someone susceptible to that virus, who then transfers the microorganism to his or her own eyes or nose; or (2) by virus-contaminated droplets sprayed into the air when an infected person sneezes, which are then inhaled by someone susceptible to that virus.

About the only thing everyone seems to agree on is that kissing someone with a cold—even kissing on the mouth and soul-kissing—rarely spreads the virus to susceptible people. Even sneezing and coughing are unlikely routes for spreading cold viruses, experts maintain. This is because cold viruses live in the cells of the nasal passages and are shed through secretions from the nose. Sneezes and coughs primarily contain secretions from the mouth and throat, not the nose (though, understandably, few healthy people would feel comfortable sitting near someone with a cold who is coughing and sneezing).

## IS IT HAND DELIVERED...

The case for hand-to-hand spread of colds is strongly supported by research conducted at the University of Virginia in Charlottesville by Dr. Jack Gwaltney, Jr., and Dr. J. Owen Hendley. Their studies seem to show that cold viruses are spread through hand-to-hand contact with people who have colds, or by touching surfaces that have been contaminated with cold virus, followed by "self-inoculation"—touching the virus-contaminated hand to the nose or eyes (cold viruses do not live in the eyes, but the tear ducts drain into the nose, providing easy passage for cold viruses). Since people commonly touch their faces several times an hour, it is easy to see how such self-inoculation can occur.

Drs. Gwaltney and Hendley tested various possible methods of transmission. For three days and nights, they housed people with colds caused by a particular virus in the same room with people susceptible to that virus. Chicken wire between them prevented any hand contact, but the healthy people were exposed to small droplets released by the cold sufferers when they talked or coughed. Another group of susceptible people were exposed to larger droplets expelled when cold-infected subjects sitting at the same small table coughed, sneezed, or talked. Finally, a third group of susceptibles had direct hand-to-hand contact with contaminated secretions from cold sufferers and then touched their own noses and eyes. None of the ten people exposed to small aerosol particles got sick, and only one of the twelve exposed to large aerosol particles caught the same cold. But in the group with hand-to-hand contact, eleven out of fifteen came down with the donors' colds.

In a later study, Drs. Gwaltney and Hendley demonstrated a high rate of cold virus transmission through the handles of ceramic coffee cups. Microbiologists have shown that cold viruses can live for hours on inanimate objects like door knobs or telephone receivers, especially if they remain moist.

## ...OR PROPELLED THROUGH THE AIR?

The competing theory that colds are spread though the air by inhaling contaminated droplets released by cold victims is espoused by Dr. Elliot Dick, professor of preventive medicine at the University of Wisconsin Medical School in Madison. He and his colleagues studied groups of men with colds who played poker for twelve hours with healthy men susceptible to the viruses involved. Half the healthy men were fitted with neck collars or arm braces that kept them from touching their faces. Thus, the only way the restrained players could catch a cold was through the air.

In three of the experiments, the infection rate among those wearing restraints was 55 percent and the rate among the unrestrained players was only slightly higher, at 66 percent. However, in a fourth experiment, Dr. Dick separated the sick men and the healthy men. First, he got the men with colds to contaminate the playing cards and chips with nasal secretions. Then in a separate room twelve new healthy, unrestrained volunteers played poker with these contaminated cards and chips and were told to repeatedly touch their eyes and noses during the game. Not one of the twelve caught a cold.

According to Dr. Dick, this series of experiments strongly supports aerosol transmission of cold viruses and seriously questions their spread through hand-to-hand-to-nose contact. It is also possible that both theories are correct; different cold viruses may be spread most efficiently by different mechanisms, and the most efficient mode may depend on the circumstances. Since contaminated droplets do not travel far, you would have to be fairly close to an infected person to catch his or her cold.

## WHY MORE COLDS IN WINTER?

Actually, the annual "cold season" begins in late August and peaks in September and October. That's when children return to school and once again come into close contact with one another's germs. The children, in turn, bring their colds home and can transmit them to preschool siblings, Mom and Dad, and anyone else in the household who might be susceptible to the viruses involved. Sending a child to school with a cold will not hurt the child, but it will increase the chance of spreading the illness to other children and, in turn, to their families.

Once outdoor temperatures drop enough to require indoor heating, the heat dries the air, which in turn dries the mucous membranes in the nose and throat, making them more susceptible to viral infection. Even outdoor air in winter is much drier than in summer, since cold air cannot hold as much moisture as warm air.

Making the buildings that we live and work and go to school in "tight" to save energy can only aggravate the problem of viral transmission by cutting down on the circulation of fresh, uncontaminated air.

A second peak of colds occurs in early spring. No one has a very good explanation for this phenomenon, but clearly one cannot blame having to endure cold weather for the increase in colds in winter. Besides, being exposed to low temperatures, having wet feet, failing to wear a hat or gloves, and other such motherly concerns have been demonstrated *not* to increase people's chances of getting a cold.

## HOW YOU GET THE FLU

The flu spreads much more readily than a cold, primarily moving directly from person to person via virus-contaminated airborne droplets released by coughs and sneezes and even normal conversation. The illness also can be spread through hands and inanimate objects. Like cold viruses, flu viruses can live for a brief time— about one to three hours—on an infected person's hands and on objects handled by contaminated hands.

Also like colds, flu can be transmitted by people who have not yet developed symptoms. The incubation period—the time between becoming infected with the virus and knowing you are ill—is one to three days, and during that time you can spread the virus to someone else. So trying to contain the illness by isolating flu victims is rarely a successful strategy. Once flu symptoms develop, you remain contagious for another three to five days. All told, then, you can be a vector for flu virus for about one week.

---

### Why Do You Get So Many Colds?

Some people, for both internal and external reasons, are more hospitable to cold viruses than others. The following factors can help you understand why you may be a likely candidate for a cold.

**Age:** Infants and young children get the most colds, up to 10 a year, because they are immune to few, if any, cold viruses. The older you get, the fewer colds you are likely to have to endure, unless you are frequently exposed to small children who carry cold viruses.

**Sex:** Women get more colds than men do, probably because women usually spend more time in the company of children.

**Menstrual cycle:** Women are more likely to catch a cold around the time of ovulation than at other times in the menstrual cycle.

**Income:** Low-income families, who often live in close quarters, get more colds than people in middle- and upper-income families, who are better able to keep their distance from one another.

**Stress:** Highly stressed individuals are more susceptible to colds than people with calmer temperaments, perhaps because undue stress weakens the immune system and prompts many people to neglect wholesome living habits.

**Smoking:** Smokers may not get more colds than nonsmokers, but they do suffer more severe symptoms. The children of smokers are more susceptible to all kinds of respiratory ailments, including colds, pneumonia, and asthma.

**Personality type:** Shy people seem to suffer more severe colds than those with more outgoing personalities.

**Immune function:** People with illnesses that tax or weaken their immune system or who must take medication that suppresses the immune response are more likely than others to catch colds.

# PREVENTING COLDS

## NO VACCINE AND PROBABLY NO VITAMINS

The ideal preventive of infectious diseases—a vaccine—remains a futuristic and, many experts say, highly doubtful notion when it comes to colds. There are just too many viruses and viral variants involved to produce an effective vaccine against all or even the most prevalent among them. About 200 strains of viruses from eight different viral groups can cause the common cold. Other less direct preventives, like administering interferon or taking large doses of vitamin C, have not proved effective in preventing infection, although vitamin C can sometimes lessen the symptoms and shorten the duration of a cold (see p. 21).

Thanks to the promotion of vitamin C by the late Linus Pauling, twice a Nobel laureate (though not a physician or even a biologist), many people have become true believers in the ability of daily supplements of vitamin C to keep colds at bay. Unfortunately, well-designed scientific studies have not borne out the preventive role of even hefty doses of vitamin C. In those studies, people who took vitamin C got sick just as often as those who didn't, although the supplement users tended to have fewer symptoms and recover more quickly.

Keep in mind, too, that large doses of vitamin C are not entirely without risk. Most of the vitamin C you might take is excreted in the urine after passing through your kidneys. Some people who take thousands of milligrams of vitamin C may be at risk of developing kidney stones, an extraordinarily painful condition that typically lands people in the hospital. Also, the resulting acidity of the urine can be highly irritating, sometimes mimicking the discomfort caused by a urinary tract infection.

Once you feel the first inklings of an incipient cold, taking large doses of vitamin C (perhaps 1,000 milligrams every 4 to 6 hours for a day or two) may suppress cold symptoms and perhaps shorten the illness. Studies suggest that this tactic helps about one-third of those coming down with a cold. But it doesn't work for all colds, even in those people it usually helps.

## EAT INFECTION-FIGHTING FOODS

Researchers have identified a number of substances in common foods that can help to ward off infectious illnesses. To maximize your resistance, include these foods in your daily diet: any member of the cabbage family—broccoli, cauliflower, mustard greens, kale, Brussels sprouts, and all forms of cabbage; garlic and onions; citrus fruits, berries, tomatoes, and peppers; and zinc-rich foods like wheat germ, whole grains, seafood, and meat.

## DON'T SMOKE

Of course, this is a good idea even if preventing colds is not your concern. Smoking paralyzes the cilia, the tiny hairs that line the respiratory tract and are a first-line defense against infection. The cilia help to sweep out debris, including virus-contaminated mucus. Passive smoking, too, can increase your risk of infection. Infants and young children exposed to passive smoke are more likely to develop pneumonia and asthma.

## REDUCE STRESS

Have you ever noticed that you're most likely to come down with a cold when you're about to leave on a trip or vacation, or when you're rushing to meet a deadline, or when you're cramming for a big exam? Dr. Sheldon Cohen, a psychologist at Carnegie-Mellon University in Pittsburgh, showed that people who test out as having the highest stress level are twice as likely to catch a cold as those on the lowest end of the stress continuum. So, relax! Try to reduce your stress level through regular exercise, meditation, yoga, T'ai chi, listening to relaxation tapes or sedating music, or any other harmless activity that can calm you down.

Learn to pace yourself. Keep balance in your life, allowing ample time for pleasure, regular aerobic exercise, relaxation, friends, fun, changes of scenery, and vacations from work or daily routines.

## DROWN THEM OUT

Just as you would flush a toilet to rid it of waste, it also helps to flush out your body to cleanse it of potentially infectious organisms like cold viruses. Drink plenty of fluids, especially those that hydrate the body—that is, fluids that are free of caffeine, alcohol, excessive sugar or salt. That leaves water as the best thing to drink. Other useful beverages include decaffeinated coffee and tea, caffeine-free herb teas, seltzer, club soda, mineral water, and diluted fruit juices. The liquid helps to keep mucous membranes moist, enabling them to trap cold viruses and dispose of them before they can infect your cells. This is especially important during the winter months, when both indoor and outdoor air are much drier. One of the best weapons yet invented to ward off respiratory viruses may be the quart-sized sports bottle; fill it with water, carry it around with you, and sip from it all day long.

Close contact with potentially infected people is but one reason why colds spread so easily in winter or when you take a long plane trip. Another is extreme dehydration—especially the drying out of those nasal passages, your first line of defense against cold viruses. Homes, cars, and workplaces that are heated in winter typically have humidity levels of 20 to 30 percent. And airplane air at any time of year is comparable in dryness to the Sahara Desert. At home, you might try humidifying the air at night with a steam vaporizer (cold-mist humidifiers often foster the growth and dispersal of infectious organisms and allergens). Another strategy that some people find helpful is to program the thermostat so that the heat is off when you sleep and doesn't come up until you get up and can start drinking again. But at work and during travel, your only option is to keep yourself moist from within by drinking lots and lots of plain fluids—eight ounces for every hour of travel is a good benchmark for maintaining decent hydration.

## AIR THEM OUT

A further problem in enclosed spaces is the enforced breathing of recycled and potentially contaminated air. Studies by Dr. Dick suggest that good ventilation can help disperse nasty cold (and flu) viruses. The "old wives" who spun tales may have known this when they recommended opening the bedroom window at least a little while you sleep. At home or work, a forced-air ventilation system can help, if it is kept in working order. If the air is heated by radiators or an electric baseboard, consider using fans to help keep it circulating. On a plane, of course, there's nothing you can do to cleanse the air, which makes keeping yourself well hydrated all the more important. Those who believe in the protective value of vitamin C (despite the lack of scientific evidence) might also try taking about 1,000 milligrams of vitamin C just before a plane trip and perhaps a second dose after landing.

## USE DISPOSABLE TISSUES

When you have a cold, it is far better to use disposable tissues than a handkerchief, which can keep your hands perpetually contaminated with the infectious virus. Dispose of used tissues promptly by discarding them in a manner that makes rehandling them unnecessary. The use of paper towels, paper cups, and liquid soaps in the bathroom may also help reduce the spread of colds within the household.

Kimberly-Clark developed facial tissues impregnated with an

antiviral compound, and Dr. Dick of Wisconsin showed that their use could dramatically reduce the spread of colds. But attempts by the company to market these tissues, which cost about three times as much as ordinary tissues, failed. Consumers, it seems, would rather sniff and save than contain their colds.

## WASH THOSE HANDS

Regardless of who may be correct about how colds are spread (see p. 13), it seems wise to follow the prevalent advice: wash your hands often, especially if you are working or living with someone with a cold. Change towels and washcloths often and wash them in hot water; better yet, give each person in the household his or her own color-coded hand towel and washcloth.

Unless you have just washed your hands, keep them away from your nose and eyes. According to B. Burton, a nurse and infection control specialist at the National Jewish Center for Immunology and Respiratory Medicine in Denver, Colorado, "The average person touches his face within the area of the eyes, nose and mouth about once every 20 minutes."

Of course, if you are the one with the cold, it's only common courtesy to wash your hands often, especially after blowing your nose, and to keep your hands to yourself. If you want to show really good manners, when you have a cold and must greet someone, refrain from the conventional handshake. Apologize and explain that you'd rather keep your cold to yourself.

It is also time to question whether it is good manners to cover coughs and sneezes with your hands. To reduce the risk of spreading your illness to others, it would be better to keep your hands away from your face and instead turn your head away.

## KEEP SURFACES CLEAN

Don't forget: cold viruses and other infectious organisms often live for hours on inanimate objects, especially those that remain moist. If possible, try to avoid using objects like telephones, pens and pencils, and keyboards that have been used by someone with a cold. However, cold experts say that keyboards, door knobs, telephones, and other commonly touched surfaces can be rendered germ-free by wiping them with a cotton ball dipped in rubbing alcohol or by using an alcohol wipe. Also effective for cleaning potentially contaminated surfaces is a household disinfectant containing 0.1 percent phenylphenol and 68 percent alcohol (e.g. Lysol Disinfectant Spray), available in drugstores and supermarkets.

What do you do, though, about surfaces at work, in public places, or in other people's homes? Few would feel comfortable walking around with a disinfectant spray, spritzing door knobs, handlebars, cup handles, etc. before touching them. Some use paper towels to open doors, say, in a public rest room. Others to whom it is extremely important to avoid a cold might follow a practice popular in Japan of wearing a disposable mask over the nose and mouth when out in crowded public places. It's not exactly glamorous, but it might help to keep you healthy. For travelers and others who often use public telephones and who want to keep the risk of infection to a minimum, individually packaged alcohol wipes might be used to clean the receiver.

# PREVENTING THE FLU

When it comes to avoiding influenza, you have fewer environmental options. Flu viruses can spread very easily from person to person via contaminated droplets released into the air when someone harboring live flu virus speaks, coughs, or sneezes. Since the flu virus incubates in your body for a day or two before symptoms develop, sometimes the flu is spread to others before a person even knows he or she is getting sick. Certainly once those classic flu symptoms start, the considerate victim will high-tail it home immediately and avoid even casual personal contacts for the first three or four days of the illness.

## VACCINES TO THE RESCUE

But unlike colds, there are many fewer viruses that cause the flu, and despite their fickle nature, it is possible to prevent the flu by an annual vaccine taken weeks before the flu season. Researchers worldwide monitor the changes in the flu virus, and before each flu season, manufacturers are usually able to produce a revised vaccine that incorporates protection against the newest virus variants.

Chances are you've heard recommendations that flu vaccine be given annually to people over sixty-five, to people like the police and firefighters who perform essential services, and to anyone with a chronic illness like heart or lung disease or an immune deficiency that can turn even a mild flu into a deadly disease (see Box 2 on pp. 31–34 for the full set of recommendations). Being a younger, healthy person in a "nonessential" occupation, perhaps you think the flu vaccine is not for you. Perhaps you view a bout with the flu as a mini-vacation, an excuse to escape from your normal duties. Or perhaps friends told you that when they took the vaccine, they got a reaction that was almost as bad as the flu itself.

Well, if any of these "perhapses" applies to you, think again. Anyone, regardless of age or health status, is entitled to and can benefit from flu vaccine, assuming the person can afford it. The public health recommendations about who should be immunized are designed to protect those at highest risk of suffering life-threatening complications from the flu. They were issued primarily because there simply isn't enough flu vaccine to go around if every young, healthy person got the shot too. But times are changing, and new technologies and an increased number of vaccine producers have helped to expand the supply, which would no doubt grow larger if the demand for the vaccine were greater.

Having the flu is no fun, and chances are you'll feel too ill to do any of those housebound projects you've been meaning to get around to. If you can't afford to be flattened by the flu for a week or more, and debilitated for weeks longer, you'd be wise to get the vaccine in October or early November *every year*. Waiting until the flu hits your community is not wise; it usually takes two to three weeks after you receive the vaccine for your body to build up an immunity to the viruses. However, public health officials advise that high-risk individuals who were not previously immunized should get the vaccine even if a flu outbreak is already under way.

Vaccine side effects have been greatly exaggerated. *It is biologically impossible to get the flu from the vaccine* because the viruses in the vaccine are dead and incapable of invading and reproducing in your cells. All they can do is rev up your body's immune system and prompt it to produce antibodies that would knock out the live flu viruses should you encounter them. If you do suffer a flulike reaction from the vaccine, chances are you are extremely susceptible to the viruses the vaccine is designed to protect against. If you were unprotected and contracted the flu from one of those live viruses, you would undoubtedly become extremely ill. It's better by far to have a brief flulike vaccine reaction than the full-blown flu. The most common vaccine reaction is not illness at all but rather some minor redness and soreness at the site of the injection that goes away in a day or two.

There are, however, a few people who should not take flu vaccine. Since the vaccine is produced from viruses that are grown in eggs, those with a severe allergy to eggs should avoid it. People who are already suffering from an infectious illness had best let themselves recover before getting a flu shot. The vaccine can be given safely to very young children, although they commonly get more side effects than adults do. Babies over age six months who have ailments that place them in a high-risk category for serious complications of the flu can be given a so-called split-virus vaccine to minimize side effects.

Flu vaccine is effective, but it is not perfect. In general it is 70 to 90 percent effective in preventing the flu that is going around that year. Unfortunately, it is more effective in younger people than in the elderly, who most need its protection. Also, it has a time-limited benefit. Even if the flu viruses don't change from one year to the next, the immunity induced by the vaccine only lasts about one year. So you would need to get an annual shot no matter how the virus behaves.

## ANTIVIRAL AGENTS SOMETIMES HELP

For people who cannot take flu vaccine or who failed to get vaccine protection in time and face a high risk of serious complications from the flu, there are two antiviral drugs—amantadine hydrochloride (Symmetrel) and rimantidine hydrochloride (Flumadine)—that can help to prevent infection by the type A flu virus, the most deadly one. These drugs are also helpful for people who took the vaccine but need extra protection, such as elderly people with heart or lung disease.

The drugs prevent type A flu viruses (but not type B viruses) from multiplying in the body. They are about 75 to 80 percent effective in preventing type A influenza, the type of flu that results in the most serious complications. However, to be effective, they must be taken daily before a flu outbreak begins and throughout the entire flu season since, unlike the vaccine, they have no lasting effect. In addition to their preventive value, the drugs may help shorten the course of an attack of type A influenza among people who should have been vaccinated but weren't.

The drugs have some side effects that unfortunately are more frequent in people over sixty-five, the group most in need of protection. Typical side effects involve the central nervous system: difficulty sleeping, tremulousness, depression or confusion. However, these effects are usually mild and often go away while the medication is still being taken.

---

### Who Should Get Flu Vaccine

The Centers for Disease Control and Prevention, a division of the U.S. Public Health Service, strongly recommends that certain people be vaccinated against influenza every year before the flu season begins. Children twelve years of age and younger should be given only the so-called split-virus vaccine. Children under nine years of age who have not been previously vaccinated should get two doses of split-virus vaccine, with a one-month gap between them and with the second dose given before December. Although the best time for vaccination is between October 15 and November 15, high-risk individuals who were not previously immunized may still benefit from vaccination even after a flu outbreak has begun in their communities.

Charges for a flu shot are now fully reimbursable for everyone covered by Medicare. The vaccine is also offered for a minimal fee at many public health clinics and health maintenance organizations (HMOs) and it is increasingly being offered free of charge to employees of large companies. Check with your local health department or your company's medical department or benefits office. The vaccine is also available for a fee from many private physicians.

The current U.S. Public Health Service recommendations for flu vaccination are as follows:

### Groups at High Risk for Serious Influenza Complications

- Every person aged 65 and older.
- Infants over 6 months of age and all children and adults with chronic heart or lung disease, cystic fibrosis, a chronic metabolic disorder like diabetes, kidney disease, anemia, or severe asthma.
- People of any age with cancer or an immunological disorder (including HIV infection) or those on medications that suppress immunity and lower the body's resistance to infection.
- All residents of nursing homes and other chronic-care facilities, particularly those with long-term health problems.
- Children and teenagers (aged 6 months to 18 years) who are on long-term aspirin therapy (they may be at risk of developing a life-threatening condition called Reye's syndrome should they get the flu while taking aspirin).

### Groups That Can Transmit Influenza to High-Risk Persons

- Physicians, nurses, and other personnel who work in a hospital, outpatient facility, nursing home, or chronic-care facility and have contact with high-risk patients in all age groups, including infants.

- Health-care workers and volunteers who provide in-home care to high-risk persons.
- Household members, including children, of anyone who is at high risk for serious flu complications.

### Other Groups

While they are not covered by official public health recommendations, other people who might consider taking an annual flu shot include:

- People like the police and firefighters who provide essential community services.
- Students, teachers, day-care personnel, and others who work in institutional settings.
- Pregnant women who have other medical conditions that might increase their risk of flu complications. If possible, the vaccine should be administered after the first 3 months of pregnancy. However, vaccination of high-risk women should not be delayed if they will still be in the first trimester when the flu season begins.
- Foreign travelers who expect to be in tropics at any time of the year or in the southern hemisphere during April through September, when the flu season hits there. Pretravel vaccination with the previous season's vaccine is especially important for those in high-risk categories.
- Any person who wants to reduce his or her chances of getting the flu. Only cost and vaccine availability limit the ability of every young, healthy person to take an annual flu shot.

### Who Should Not Be Vaccinated

- People with extreme allergic reactions to eggs, since the virus

used in the vaccine is grown in eggs and the vaccine can contain
minute amounts of egg protein.

- People with fever-causing illnesses, who should wait until they
  recover to take a flu shot.

## THE FICKLE FLU VIRUS

The viruses that cause influenza are genetically unstable. They
change both gradually and abruptly, and each change may enable
the virus to skirt around previously acquired immunity, invade the
respiratory tract, and cause the flu. This genetic instability is why
people can get influenza over and over again, why they get it some
years and not others, why some attacks make them much sicker
than others, and why it's necessary to get a new flu shot every year
for maximum protection.

The gradual changes in the virus, called antigenic *drift*, may or
may not be enough to override most people's immunity to it. But
when the abrupt changes known as antigenic *shift* occur, large num-
bers of people—and sometimes the entire population—have no
protection. Such shifts usually result in worldwide epidemics, or
pandemics, and, when they involve type A flu viruses, they are often highly lethal.

Type A flu viruses have two major antigens on their surface called
H and N (the "H" stands for hemagglutinin and the "N" for
neuraminidase). When they encounter a person's immune system,
these antigens trigger the production of antibodies that protect the
person against the viral infection. When major changes occur in H

and/or N, most people have no preexisting antibody protection, and so they are susceptible to an invasion by the new form of the virus. The following table shows the major shifts that have occurred in the type A influenza virus during this century. The pandemics are usually named for the area where the virus was first isolated.

There is evidence that during the last decade of the nineteenth century, a type A virus very similar to the H2N2 Asian flu virus prevailed, and that during the first seventeen years of the twentieth century a virus similar to the H3N2 Hong Kong virus was the primary troublemaker.

The Spanish flu A-H1N1 virus that first appeared in 1918 lingered in the population until 1957, when the Asian virus, A-H2N2, emerged and supplanted it. However, in 1977 a virus reappeared that was virtually identical to the A-H1N1 that had circulated at least until 1950. Most people born before 1950 had immunity to the 1977 virus, but those who were younger or who had missed being exposed to the original cause of Spanish flu had no natural protection, and many became very ill.

In 1992, the type A virus genetically rearranged some of its attire, but did not do a total costume switch. A variant known as Beijing arose, an A-H3N2 virus that was a kissing cousin of the A-H3N2 virus that caused the Hong Kong flu in 1968. Thus, many people had at least a partial immunity to it because they had encountered its close relative in the past. In the 1994–95 flu season, yet another A-H3N2 virus called Shandong was a leading troublemaker.

What will come along next is anybody's guess. But the nation's flu watchers are always on guard, and as soon as any new variant arises that causes a significant outbreak of influenza anywhere in the world, the manufacturers of flu vaccine will be ready to add it to their mix.

### TABLE 3: FLU PANDEMICS

| Year | Name of Pandemic | Viral Type | Mortality |
|------|------------------|------------|-----------|
| 1918–19 | Spanish flu | A-H1N1 | 500,000 deaths in the U.S. 20 million deaths worldwide |
| 1957–58 | Asian flu | A-H2N2 | 70,000 deaths in the U.S. |
| 1968–69 | Hong Kong flu | A-H3N2 | 34,000 deaths in the U.S. |

# TREATING COLDS AND FLU

$A$sk twenty people what they do for themselves when they catch a cold and chances are you'll get twenty different answers. That's because there is no cure for a cold, only treatments to suppress the symptoms. The proverbial wisdom still applies: Treat a cold and it will be gone in a week; don't treat it and it will last seven days!

Most of the treatments used today are only slightly more effective, in fact, than the cold remedies of yore. The ancient Chinese recommended eating snakeskin. British soldiers advised wrapping a fresh-off-the-foot sock around the throat at night. Sir William Osler, a famous English physician of the early twentieth century, suggested hanging a hat on the bedpost, getting into bed, and drinking whiskey until you see two hats. The treatment did little for the cold, but perhaps made the patient less aware of his discomfort.

Despite the many advertised promises of "fast, *fast*, FAST relief" from a plethora of cold and flu products, chances are you'll recover just as quickly if you took none of them and instead applied some of the time-honored home remedies on pages 53–54 and perhaps one or two of the "natural" remedies on pages 55–58. Or, you could follow the lead of a British medical officer who said he never takes medicine: "If I get a cold, I treat it with the contempt it deserves." And if mental ostracism does not do the trick, time will.

There are some cautionary tales when trying to cope with upper respiratory infections. Most important, perhaps, is the questionable wisdom of treating the symptoms. Since symptoms like fever and cough represent the body's efforts to cure itself, some practitioners say these signs of healing should not be suppressed unless they introduce further threats to health. Unless fever goes above, say, 102°F and a cough disrupts sleep, it may be best to let them run their course.

---

### How a Cold Progresses

It may give you little comfort to know that most of the symptoms of a cold are caused, not by the cold virus attacking you, but by your body's immune system attacking the virus. In other words, you feel worse because you're getting better.

**Enter the virus:** In a sneak attack you have no way of detecting, cold viruses enter the upper respiratory tract through the nose or are transported there through the eyes.

**The viral attack:** Viruses that do not get entrapped and flushed out

by the tiny hairs and mucus that line the nasal passages can pen-
etrate the layer of mucus and attach themselves to cells in the throat,
where they multiply and disperse throughout the nose and throat.
At this point, you still have no reason to suspect an impending cold.

**Body cells fight back:** Within an hour of the viral attack, throat
cells injured by the virus launch a counterattack, releasing chemi-
cals that trigger inflammation and attract white blood cells to fight
off the infection. As a result, the tissues become red and begin to
swell, though you probably are still unaware of what lies ahead.

**Reinforcements arrive:** White blood cells called macrophages—
the "gobblers" of the immune system—arrive to engulf the invading
viruses. This attack triggers the release of several infection-fighting
proteins.

**Symptoms blossom:** About a day after the throat cells become infected, the developing inflammation causes a sore throat and the
defensive proteins that are released induce chills and muscle aches.
These proteins also combine with blood in the nose to cause nasal
swelling—that unmistakable feeling of congestion—and a runny
nose. The excess mucus, in turn, can trigger a cough.

**Symptoms subside:** The immune system begins to get the upper
hand within 3 to 7 days of the viral invasion. Inflammation sub-
sides, mucus production gradually returns to normal, and you start
to feel significantly better.

## COLD/FLU MEDICINES: COMPONENTS
## AND CAUTIONS

As if consumers weren't already confused enough by the hundreds
of cold/flu remedies, every year several dozen new products are
introduced in hopes that they will capture a significant portion of
the more than $1.4 billion over-the-counter market. Most are
slightly altered versions of already existing products. Many contain
a mix of ingredients, only some of which may be useful while others may be counterproductive.

If any medications are taken at all, experts advise that single-ingredient products be used, chosen to counter the most bothersome
of your symptoms. When treating a cold, less is best. *The more ingredients you take, the more likely you will experience adverse side effects that
may actually make you feel worse.* Keep in mind, too, that as a cold
progresses, the symptoms change, and so should the treatment.

Pregnant women should not take any medication without check-
ing first with their physicians. The elderly, too, should exercise caution, since they are more likely to experience toxic side effects from
both over-the-counter and prescribed drugs. Also, anyone with a
chronic health problem, from heart disease to glaucoma, and anyone taking prescribed medication, including psychotherapeutic
drugs, should check with a physician before taking any over-the-
counter cold/flu product.

Whatever drug you choose, there is no inherent advantage in
paying more for heavily advertised "name" brands; generic or store-

brand versions will work just as well (or as poorly). Here is what you might find in a cold/flu medicine.

**Active ingredients:** These are the substances that are supposed to have a direct effect on symptoms. They include analgesics (pain-killers) and antipyretics (fever reducers), decongestants, cough suppressants, expectorants, and antihistamines.

**Inactive ingredients:** These include substances like alcohol that give the medicine form and texture, flavoring and coloring agents, stabilizers, sugar, and caffeine (often added to counter the drowsiness induced by antihistamines, but not too helpful if what you need most is sleep).

**Analgesics and antipyretics:** The common painkillers—aspirin, acetaminophen, and ibuprofen—play two roles. They relieve headaches and muscle aches and they reduce fever. If a product containing any of these is used, additional pain or fever medication should not be taken. Of the three, acetaminophen is least likely to cause stomach upset. Before taking aspirin or ibuprofen, it is wise to eat something. Aspirin has been shown to increase viral shedding (and thus may help to spread the cold to others) and it may also prolong the infection. Remember, too, that fever is one of the body's main weapons against infectious organisms, so unless it is very high (say, above 102°F in an adult), you may want to let it run its course.

**Decongestants:** These help to relieve upper respiratory congestion (stuffy nose and sinuses) by shrinking blood vessels and reducing swelling in the nasal passages. But relief comes at a price. Oral decongestants can cause dry mouth, agitation, insomnia, increased heart rate, and raised blood pressure. Pseudoephedrine is the most popular decongestant used in oral medications. Phenylpropanolamine (PPA), the most common ingredient in diet drugs, is also often used as an oral decongestant, but it is more likely than pseudoephedrine to cause a steep rise in blood pressure. Oral decongestants may interfere with restful sleep and result in daytime fatigue. Limit their use to one week to avoid a rebound reaction—an increase in congestion and dependency on the product. Fewer side effects are associated with topical decongestants in nose drops and nasal sprays. Effective ingredients include xylometazoline, oxymetazoline, ephredrine, and phenylephrine. However, nose drops and sprays should not be used longer than three days; longer use can cause a rebound reaction.

**Cough suppressants:** These products, also known as antitussives, are used to suppress an irritative, dry cough. Experts recommend that they be reserved for coughs that disrupt sleep. Lingering coughs that interfere with a person's waking life are best treated with home remedies like ample fluids, cough drops, and lozenges. The most popular cough-suppressant product is dextromethorphan. Others deemed effective are chlophendianol and codeine (a prescription drug that is sleep-inducing and can be habit-forming).

**Expectorants:** When a cough is "productive"—sputum-producing—it is consider a "good" cough that is cleansing the breathing tubes of excess mucus and potentially infectious microorganisms. The goal is not to suppress such a cough but rather to liquefy and loosen the phlegm so that it is more easily coughed up. This is the role of expectorants. Expectorants may also help to loosen up a "tight-chested" nonproductive cough that results from an accumulation of secretions so thick they cannot be coughed up. The only expectorant approved as safe and effective for over-the-counter use is guaifenesin. Though it may seem counterproductive to take a product that contains both an expectorant and a cough suppressant, the combination may be helpful when taken before bedtime if a productive cough frequently interrupts sleep.

**Antihistamines:** These products are designed to counter the symptoms of allergies by blocking the effects of histamine. Histamines play almost no role in colds and flu, but antihistamines have a potent drying effect, which has prompted their widespread use in products designed to stop the runny nose that is the hallmark of the early stages of a cold. However, this is one ingredient experts say should be avoided by cold and flu sufferers because it can thicken secretions in the chest and sinuses, making them harder to expel and setting the stage for a secondary infection. The antihistamines approved for over-the-counter use also cause drowsiness, adding to the fatigue induced by a cold and making driving or operating machinery very hazardous. Other side effects may include blurred vision, dry mouth, constipation, and urine retention. The most commonly used antihistamines in over-the-counter products are chlorpheniramine, triprolidine, brompheniramine, and doxylamine.

## TABLE 4: WHAT SHOULD YOU TAKE FOR RELIEF?

Combination medicines for colds and flu are rarely a good idea because you end up taking drugs you don't need and may not get enough of the medications that could actually help you to feel better. Instead, an advisory panel to the Food and Drug Administration (FDA) has recommended that cold symptoms be treated individually. You will notice that antihistamines are not on this list. Although they do dry up nasal secretions, antihistamines should be used with caution in treating symptoms of a respiratory infection because they can dry out mucous membranes and thicken secretions in the sinuses and bronchial passages, which may set the stage for further congestion and possibly a bacterial infection.

| Symptom | What Can Help | Ingredients That Work |
|---|---|---|
| Headache, muscle ache, fever | pain reliever, fever reducer | aspirin, acetaminophen, ibuprofen |
| Nasal congestion | oral decongestant | pseudoephedrine |
| Acute nasal congestion (before sleep and upon awakening) | nasal spray | phenylephrine, oxymetazoline xylometazoline |
| Productive or "tight" cough | expectorant | guaifenesin |
| Dry cough that disrupts sleep | cough suppressant | dextromethorphan, codeine*, chlophendianol |
| Sore throat | medicated lozenges or sprays | phenol compounds, benzocaine, hexylresorcinol, menthol |

* Available only by prescription

# TABLE 5: WHAT'S IN THAT COMBINATION PRODUCT?

In general, experts in infectious disease advise against taking combination products. You may end up taking medication you don't need and not enough of what would really help, and you will increase your chances of experiencing undesirable side effects. But if you decide to go with a combination product, here is what you will get.

| Product | Analgesic | Decongestant | Cough Suppressant | Expectorant | Antihistamine |
|---|---|---|---|---|---|
| Actifed (tablet) | | pseudoephedrine | | | triprolidine |
| Actifed Plus (tablet) | acetaminophen | pseudoephedrine | | | triprolidine |
| Actifed Sinus Daytime/Nighttime (tablet) | acetaminophen | pseudoephedrine | | | diphenhydramine (night only) |
| Advil Cold & Sinus (caplet) | ibuprofen | pseudoephedrine | | | |
| Alka-Seltzer Plus Cold (tablet) | aspirin | phenylpropanolamine | | | chlorpheniramine |
| Alka-Seltzer Plus Cold and Cough (tablet) | aspirin | phenylpropanolamine | dextromethorphan | | chlorpheniramine |
| Alka-Seltzer Plus Night-time Cold | aspirin | phenylpropanolamine | dextromethorphan | | brompheniramine |
| Bayer Select Chest Cold (caplet) | acetaminophen | | dextromethorphan | | |
| Bayer Select Flu Relief (caplet) | acetaminophen | pseudoephedrine | dextromethorphan | | chlorpheniramine |
| Bayer Select Head Cold (caplet) | acetaminophen | pseudoephedrine | | | |
| Bayer Select Head & Chest Cold (caplet) | acetaminophen | pseudoephedrine | dextromethorphan | guaifenesin | |
| Bayer Select Night Time Cold (caplet) | acetaminophen | pseudoephedrine | dextromethorphan | | triprolidine |
| Benadryl Cold/Flu (tablet) | acetaminophen | pseudoephedrine | | | diphenhydramine |

## TABLE 5: WHAT'S IN THAT COMBINATION PRODUCT? (Continued)

| Product | Analgesic | Decongestant | Cough Suppressant | Expectorant | Antihistamine |
|---------|-----------|--------------|-------------------|-------------|---------------|
| Benadryl Decongestant (tablet, liquid) | | pseudoephedrine | | | diphenhydramine |
| Benylin Expectorant (liquid) | | | dextromethorphan | guaifenesin | |
| Cheracol Plus Cough Syrup (liquid) | | phenylpropanolamine | dextromethorphan | guaifenesin | chlorpheniramine |
| Cheracol-D (liquid) | | | dextromethorphan | guaifenesin | |
| Comtrex (tablet) | acetaminophen | pseudoephedrine | dextromethorphan | | chlorpheniramine |
| Comtrex Day-Night (night only) | acetaminophen | pseudoephedrine | dextromethorphan | | chlorpheniramine |
| Comtrex Non-Drowsy (caplet) | acetaminophen | pseudoephedrine | dextromethorphan | | |
| Contac Day & Night Cold & Flu | acetaminophen | pseudoephedrine (day and night) | dextromethorphan (day only) | | diphenhydramine (night only) |
| Contac Continuous Action (capsule) | | phenylpropanolamine | | | chlorpheniramine |
| Contac Cough & Chest Cold (liquid) | acetaminophen | pseudoephedrine | dextromethorphan | guaifenesin | |
| Contac Cough Formula (liquid) | | | dextromethorphan | guaifenesin | |
| Contac Severe Cold & Flu Non-Drowsy (caplet) | acetaminophen | pseudoephedrine | dextromethorphan | | |
| Contac Severe Cold & Flu (caplet) | acetaminophen | phenylpropanolamine | dextromethorphan | | chlorpheniramine |
| Contac Severe Cold & Flu (powder) | acetaminophen | pseudoephedrine | dextromethorphan | | chlorpheniramine |

# TABLE 5: WHAT'S IN THAT COMBINATION PRODUCT? (Continued)

| Product | acetaminophen | decongestant | dextromethorphan | guaifenesin | antihistamine |
|---|---|---|---|---|---|
| Coricidin (tablet) | acetaminophen | | | | chlorpheniramine |
| Coricidin 'D' Decongestant (tablet) | acetaminophen | phenylpropanolamine | | | chlorpheniramine |
| Dimetapp (tablet, liquid) | | phenylpropanolamine | | | brompheniramine |
| Dimetapp Cold & Flu (caplet) | acetaminophen | phenylpropanolamine | | | brompheniramine |
| Dimetapp DM Elixir (liquid) | | phenylpropanolamine | dextromethorphan | | brompheniramine |
| Dristan Cold and Flu (powder) | acetaminophen | phenylpropanolamine | | | brompheniramine |
| Dristan Cold Non-Drowsy Formula (caplet) | acetaminophen | pseudoephedrine | | | |
| Drixoral Cold & Flu (tablet) | acetaminophen | pseudoephedrine | | | dexbrompheniramine |
| 4-Way Cold Tablets (tablet) | acetaminophen | phenylpropanolamine | | | chlorpheniramine |
| Naldecon DX (liquid) | | phenylpropanolamine | dextromethorphan | guaifenesin | |
| Percogesic (tablet) | acetaminophen | | | | phenyltoloxamine |
| Robitussin Cough & Cold Liqui-Gels (capsules) | | pseudoephedrine | dextromethorphan | guaifenesin | |
| Robitussin DM (liquid) | | | dextromethorphan | guaifenesin | |
| Robitussin Maximum Strength Cough & Cold (liquid) | | pseudoephedrine | dextromethorphan | guaifenesin | |
| Robitussin PE (liquid) | | pseudoephedrine | | guaifenesin | |
| Scot-Tussin Sugar-Free DM (liquid) | | | dextromethorphan | | chlorpheniramine |
| Sinarest (tablet) | acetaminophen | pseudoephedrine | | | chlorpheniramine |
| Sinus Excedrin (tablet, caplet) | acetaminophen | pseudoephedrine | | | |
| Sudafed Cold & Cough (capsule) | acetaminophen | pseudoephedrine | dextromethorphan | guaifenesin | |
| Sudafed Cough Syrup (liquid) | | pseudoephedrine | dextromethorphan | guaifenesin | |

TABLE 5: WHAT'S IN THAT COMBINATION PRODUCT? (Continued)

| Product | Analgesic | Decongestant | Cough Suppressant | Expectorant | Antihistamine |
|---|---|---|---|---|---|
| Sudafed Plus (tablet, liquid) | | pseudoephedrine | | | chlorpheniramine |
| Sudafed Severe Cold Formula (caplet) | acetaminophen | pseudoephedrine | dextromethorphan | | |
| TheraFlu Flu and Cold (powder) | acetaminophen | pseudoephedrine | | | chlorpheniramine |
| TheraFlu Flu, Cold & Cough (powder) | acetaminophen | pseudoephedrine | dextromethorphan | | chlorpheniramine |
| TheraFlu Nighttime Flu, Cold and Cough (powder) | acetaminophen | pseudoephedrine | dextromethorphan | | chlorpheniramine |
| TheraFlu Non-Drowsy Flu, Cold & Cough (powder) | acetaminophen | pseudoephedrine | dextromethorphan | | |
| Triaminic Cold and Triaminic-12 (tablet) | | phenylpropanolamine | | | chlorpheniramine |
| Triaminic-DM Syrup (liquid) | | phenylpropanolamine | dextromethorphan | | |
| Triaminic Expectorant (liquid) | | phenylpropanolamine | | guaifenesin | |
| Triaminic Syrup (liquid) | | phenylpropanolamine | | | chlorpheniramine |
| Triaminicin (tablet) | acetaminophen | phenylpropanolamine | | | chlorpheniramine |
| Triaminicol Multi-Symptom Cold (tablet) | | phenylpropanolamine | dextromethorphan | | chlorpheniramine |
| Triaminicol Multi-Symptom Relief (liquid) | | phenylpropanolamine | dextromethorphan | | chlorpheniramine |
| Tylenol Cold and Flu No Drowsiness (powder) | acetaminophen | pseudoephedrine | dextromethorphan | | |
| Tylenol Cold Effervescent (tablet) | acetaminophen | phenylpropanolamine | | | chlorpheniramine |

## TABLE 5: WHAT'S IN THAT COMBINATION PRODUCT? (Continued)

| | | | |
|---|---|---|---|
| Tylenol Multi-Symptom Cold Medication (caplet, tablet) | acetaminophen | pseudoephedrine | dextromethorphan | chlorpheniramine |
| Tylenol No Drowsiness Cold Medication (caplet, capsule) | acetaminophen | pseudoephedrine | dextromethorphan | |
| Tylenol No Drowsiness Cold & Flu Hot Medication (powder) | acetaminophen | pseudoephedrine | dextromethorphan | |
| Tylenol Cold Night Time (liquid) | acetaminophen | pseudoephedrine, diphenhydramine | | diphenhydramine |
| Tylenol Cough (liquid) | acetaminophen | | dextromethorphan | |
| Tylenol Cough Medication with Decongestant (liquid) | acetaminophen | pseudoephedrine | dextromethorphan | |
| Tylenol No Drowsiness Flu Medication (capsule) | acetaminophen | pseudoephedrine | dextromethorphan | |

# TABLE 6: SINGLE-INGREDIENT PRODUCTS ARE PREFERABLE

The list of single-ingredient products for countering the symptoms of colds and flu is shorter but also far more useful than the list of combination products. The idea is to treat only those symptoms that are causing serious distress. Antihistamines, which help to dry nasal secretions, are not recommended because they thicken mucus and may prolong or aggravate congestion in the sinuses and chest. Many of the brand-name products listed below are also available as store brands or generic brands, and the savings can be considerable.

**Warning**: To avoid a rebound reaction, limit the use of nose drops and nasal sprays to three days.

| Product | Analgesic | Decongestant | Cough Suppressant | Expectorant |
|---|---|---|---|---|
| **ANALGESICS (PAIN RELIEVERS)** | | | | |
| Advil (tablet, caplet) | ibuprofen | | | |
| Anacin (tablet, caplet) | aspirin | | | |
| Anacin-3 (tablet) | acetaminophen | | | |
| Anacin Maximum Strength (tablet) | acetaminophen | | | |
| Ascriptin (coated tablet) buffered aspirin | | | | |
| Bayer (tablet, caplet, capsule) | aspirin | | | |
| Bufferin (tablet) | buffered aspirin | | | |
| Ecotrin (caplets, coated tablets) | aspirin | | | |
| Excedrin Extra Strength (tablet, caplet) | aspirin, acetaminophen | | | |
| Excedrin Aspirin-Free (caplet) | acetaminophen | | | |
| Motrin IB (tablet, caplet) | ibuprofen | | | |
| Norwich (tablet) | aspirin | | | |
| Nuprin (tablet, caplet) | ibuprofen | | | |
| Panex (tablet) | acetaminophen | | | |
| Tylenol (tablet) | acetaminophen | | | |

# TABLE 6: SINGLE-INGREDIENT PRODUCTS ARE PREFERAABLE (Continued)

| | | | |
|---|---|---|---|
| Vanquish (caplet) | aspirin, acetaminophen | | |

## DECONGESTANTS

| | | |
|---|---|---|
| Cenafed Syrup (liquid) | pseudoephedrine | |
| Chlcr-Trimeton Non-Drowsy 4 Hour (tablet) | pseudoephedrine | |
| Drixoral Non-Drowsy Formula | pseudoephedrine | |
| Efidac/24 (tablet) | pseudoephedrine | |
| Propagest (tablet) | pseudoephedrine | |
| Sudafed (tablet) | pseudoephedrine | |

## COUGH SUPPRESSANTS

| | | |
|---|---|---|
| Benylin Cough (liquid) | dextromethorphan | |
| Drixoral Cough (capsule) | dextromethorphan | |
| Formula 44-D (liquid) | dextromethorphan | |

## EXPECTORANTS

| | | |
|---|---|---|
| Breonesin (capsule) | | guaifenesin |
| Robituss:n (liquid) | | guaifenesin |
| Scot-Tussin Expectorant (liquid) | | guaifenesin |

## NOSE DROPS AND SPRAYS

| | | |
|---|---|---|
| Afrin (nose drops, spray) | oxymetazoline | |
| Cheracol Nasal Spray Pump (nasal spray) | oxymetazoline | |
| Dristan Long Lasting (nasal spray) | oxymetazoline | |
| Neo-Synephrine 12 Hour (nasal spray) | oxymetazoline | |
| Neo-Synephrine (nose drops, spray) | phenylephrine | |
| Otrivin (nasal spray) | xylometazoline | |
| Rhinall (nasal spray) | phenylephrine | |

**Home Remedies for Common Symptoms**

Rather than run to the pharmacy or medicine chest for every symptom of a cold or flu, consider the following practical, nondrug remedies. Often they can relieve your misery just as effectively as commercial products and spare you the expense and side effects of medication.

| Symptom | What You Can Do |
|---------|----------------|
| Chills and fever | Drink as much water and juice as possible—preferably 2 quarts a day—to counter the dehydration that causes much of the discomfort associated with fever. |
| Sore throat | Gargle with warm salt water—1/4 teaspoon to 1 teaspoon salt in 8 oz of water—to reduce the inflammation. Keep your throat moist by using a vaporizer and sucking on hard candy or fruit-juice ice cubes. |
| Stuffy nose | To thin nasal secretions, use a room vaporizer, eat hot, spicy foods, eat or drink hot broth (the proverbial chicken soup cure) and other hot drinks (e.g., tea with honey), and refrain from consuming dairy products. Use saline nose drops or nasal spray (Ocean or NaSal); you can make your own by adding 1/4 teaspoon salt and 1/4 teaspoon baking soda to 8 oz water and applying the solution with a bulb syringe. Take a long, hot shower. Try sleeping on your back with your head raised on two or three pillows. |
| Runny nose | While there is no simple remedy, it is important |

to blow your nose gingerly, with a gentle, steady pressure, to avoid pushing the infection into your ears.

**Cough**

To counter a dry, irritated cough, suck on cough drops to keep the throat moist. If the cough is tight or causes chest pain or brings up thick mucus, drink lots of liquids (see advice for Chills and fever), including hot broth, and eat hot, spicy foods to thin the secretions. A room vaporizer and a hot, steamy shower are also helpful.

**Headache**

Relieve sinus congestion by following the advice given above for treating a stuffy nose. Apply cold packs or hot packs (whichever brings more relief) to the painful area.

**Labored breathing**

Relieve wheezing due to lung congestion by consuming caffeinated beverages (coffee, tea, colas); the caffeine helps to dilate bronchial passages, making breathing easier.

**Sore nose and lips**

Irritation caused by nasal secretions and aggravated by nose blowing can be eased by a light application of petroleum jelly or an emollient lotion.

**Fatigue**

Listen to your body and rest. Extra sleep at night and a daytime nap or two are helpful. If you are well enough to exercise, it will help counter the muscle weakness that often follows an acute illness. But don't overdo it; cut back on the intensity and duration of your usual workout until your fatigue abates, then build up again gradually.

## "NATURAL" REMEDIES FOR COLDS AND FLU

The growing interest in alternative medicine—from herbs and homeopathy to meditation and imagery—has been applied with a vengeance to the treatment of colds and flu. Two facts are worth remembering: "natural" does not necessarily mean "safe"—botulinum toxin is 100 percent natural *and* extremely deadly—and none of the so-called natural remedies have been subject to well-designed clinical studies that could unequivocably establish their effectiveness (or lack of effectiveness). Still, here are some natural remedies that there is good reason to believe may have some usefulness in countering the symptoms of a cold and perhaps speeding recovery.
*Warning*: If you use any herbal remedies, be sure to treat them with the same cautions you would exercise with a "real" drug; overdosing can be just as dangerous since many plants contain potent medicinal substances.

**Chicken soup:** Popularly known as "Jewish penicillin," soup made from a fat hen was first prescribed for colds by Moses Maimonides, a rabbi and physician in twelfth-century Egypt. But it doesn't have to be made by your grandmother to make you feel better. Dr. Marvin Sackner of Mount Sinai Hospital in Miami, Florida, tested soup from a nearby delicatessen and showed that it helped to loosen and clear nasal mucus. See page 57 for my recipe for homemade chicken soup; if my grandmother were still alive, she would insist it is far more therapeutic than anything from a can or store.

**Echinacea:** This plant, a member of the daisy family, contains substances that are capable of strengthening the immune system and thus *may* help the body fight off an infection by a cold or flu virus. It should not be used on a regular basis, only when a cold or flu threatens.

**Ephedra:** This substance, from a broomlike shrub native to China, can be found in some herbal teas, including the American version, Mormon tea. Ephedra is an effective decongestant and it is the prototype for pseudoephedrine, the most popular synthetic decongestant.

**Eucalyptus:** The aromatic oil from this giant evergreen can help to relieve mucous congestion. It can be used with steam to relieve coughs and it is a component of some cough drops and cough suppressants. *Warning:* Eucalyptus should not be used for children.

**Garlic:** Allicin, the active ingredient in garlic, has antiviral properties and may also relieve aching joints (when applied to the skin). Garlic is said to act as an expectorant when consumed in a tea or used in a gargling solution.

**Ginger:** Ginger tea (made from the fresh ginger root) is a time-honored favorite for getting rid of the chills, relieving sinus and chest congestion, and countering nausea.

**Goldenseal:** This plant contains an antibiotic substance, berberine, that, like echinacea, is said to stimulate the immune system, prompting it to engulf and destroy infectious organisms. Like echinacea, it should be used only when fighting an illness like a cold or flu.

**Imagery:** Put yourself in a relaxed, meditative state and use your imagination to picture your strong and powerful immune system attacking those feeble cold and flu viruses. A study conducted by a Harvard University psychologist among thirty healthy students showed that those who used imagery in this way succeeded in boosting their immune systems, especially those elements that would fight off an invading respiratory virus.

**Oscillococcinum:** Although this homeopathic medicine is more than half a century old, it has yet to be put to a scientific test. Many swear by its ability to ward off colds and flu if taken at the first hint of an impending infection. However, anecdotal evidence does not establish facts. Homeopathy is based on a principle of dilution that in effect produces remedies with little or no active ingredients. The active ingredient in Oscillococcinum is listed as Anal barbariae hepatis et cordis extractum. It is made from many serial dilutions of an extract prepared from the heart and liver of ducks. In all likelihood, it is the user's belief in its effectiveness that occasionally results in a positive effect.

**Peppermint:** The aromatic oil of this mint plant is touted as an all-around cold fighter—a decongestant, expectorant, and cough suppressant rolled into one. A strong infusion of peppermint tea, consumed at the first sign of a cold or flu, may or may not keep it at bay but at least can alleviate the symptoms of viral infection, including cough and fever.

**Vitamin C:** Though well-designed studies have shown no benefit of even large doses of this vitamin in preventing colds, several studies have indicated that when taken at the first hint of an impending cold, it can reduce cold symptoms and shorten the duration of the infection. The recommended doses needed for an effect, though, are very high—about 500 milligrams to 1 gram every hour for the first day, and about half that amount the second day. This may result in gastric and urinary irritation in some people.

**Zinc:** Evidence for the value of zinc gluconate lozenges in countering the symptoms of a cold is mixed. Some researchers have found it helpful, while others showed no effect. Supposedly, sucking slowly on the lozenge coats the throat with zinc and stops reproduction of cold viruses. One downside: the lozenges may taste awful. Also, beware of overdosing; too much zinc can cause nausea and raise cholesterol levels.

---

### Recipe: Jane Brody's Chicken Soup
About 6 servings

When I was a child, every Friday afternoon my mother prepared delicious chicken soup with a stewing hen obtained from a live poultry market. First she "koshered" the hen by soaking and salting it. The flavorful bird was then cooked—feet, immature eggs, gizzards, and all—in a large pot with carrots, celery, onion, and garlic. You too can enjoy a dose of "Jewish penicillin" with this recipe which, despite the use of an ordinary supermarket chicken that is not koshered, comes close to tasting like the soothing soup my mother made.

**Preparation tips:** Leaving the skin and fat on the chicken while it cooks produces a tastier result, so I prepare the soup in advance, decant and cool the broth, and remove the fat. If you wish to end up with a ready-to-eat soup, remove the skin and fat pads from the chicken before cooking it. The recipe can be used to prepare clear broth or a more balanced soup with chicken and vegetables, and perhaps with cooked rice or tiny soup pasta added at the end. Either way, the finished soup can be frozen in individual portions for the days when someone in the household comes down with a cold or the flu.

**Serving suggestion:** Challah, the traditional Jewish egg bread, is a wonderful accompaniment.

3 1/2-lb whole chicken with giblets (except the liver)
12 cups (3 quarts) cold water
1 large onion, diced
2 large stalks celery, cut crosswise into 1/2-inch lengths
2 large carrots, peeled and cut crosswise into 1/2-inch lengths
3 large cloves garlic, thinly sliced crosswise
Soup greens: 2 or 3 leafy ends of celery, 3 or 4 sprigs fresh dill, 6 to
    8 sprigs parsley, and 1 bay leaf
2 teaspoons salt, preferably coarse, or to taste
1/4 teaspoon white pepper, or to taste

1. Place the whole chicken (see Preparation tips, above) and giblets in a large kettle with a lid. Add the water and turn the heat to high.

2. Add the onion, celery stalks, carrots, and garlic to the pot. Tie together the soup greens with string or wrap them in cheese-cloth and add the bundle of soup greens to the kettle. Add the salt and pepper.

3. When the water comes to a boil, reduce the heat to medium-low, partially cover the kettle, and simmer the soup for about 2 hours, or until the chicken begins to fall apart.

4. When the soup is done, remove the chicken to a large plate and set it aside to cool somewhat. Remove and discard the bundle of soup greens. Strain the broth into a large bowl. Then either chill the broth to remove the fat or pour the broth, in batches, into a fat-separating cup and then pour the defatted broth back into the kettle.

5. When the chicken is cooled enough to handle, remove and discard the skin and bones. Cut the meat into bite-sized pieces and add them to the kettle. Heat the soup thoroughly before serving it.

# COMMON CONCERNS ABOUT COLDS AND FLU

## I LOST MY VOICE, NOW WHAT?

Respiratory viruses that live in the throat can make their way to the vocal cords, causing inflammation that leads to hoarseness and occasionally to a total, albeit temporary, loss of the ability to speak audibly. Laryngitis, as this condition is called, is best treated with vocal rest. In other word, stop trying to talk and don't attempt to communicate in whispers. This only further irritates the vocal cords and prolongs the problem. Take up writing instead. Drink as much fluid as you can, avoid dairy products and smoke, humidify your bedroom with a room vaporizer, suck on soothing lozenges, and wait it out.

## WHY DON'T I FEEL BETTER?

Colds and flu don't always disappear without leaving behind a legacy that can drag on for weeks or longer. Sinus infections and ear infections are common sequels of a cold, even when the cold itself was not severe, and bronchitis or even pneumonia can follow a bout of influenza. These complications require prompt medical attention.

A lingering irritative cough is best treated by drinking as much fluid as you can, sucking on soothing lozenges, humidifying your bedroom with a room vaporizer, and perhaps taking a cough suppressant. Those with asthma may suffer an exacerbation of asthmatic symptoms, and occasionally a person who did not have asthma before may develop it as a result of a bad cold or flu.

Sometimes breathing tubes will become temporarily hypersensitive, resulting in coughing upon exposure to minor irritants like perfume or smoke. Asthma medications may be needed to relieve this condition.

Then there is the fatigue, which can drag on for weeks after any viral infection and especially after the flu. Give in to it and get extra rest.

## WHEN CAN ANTIBIOTICS HELP?

Antibiotics like penicillin, tetracycline, and sulfa drugs are potent killers of bacteria, but they have absolutely no effect against the viruses that cause colds and flu. Unless you suffer from a chronic lung disease, it is not helpful—and it could be harmful—to take antibiotics in anticipation of a possible bacterial infection.

However, since colds can set the stage for more serious bacterial infections like sinusitis, bronchitis, and otitis media (ear infection), antibiotics can then be called upon to attack the offending organisms and cure the infection. When antibiotics are prescribed, it is very important to take them according to the recommended frequency for the entire time specified by the physician. Otherwise, small pockets of bacteria may survive and return to cause another infection.

## CAN I TAKE ANYTHING FOR THE FLU?

An analgesic/antipyretic like aspirin, acetaminophen, or ibuprofen will help to reduce a raging fever and ease the muscle aches and headache that often accompany influenza. An expectorant and/or cough suppressant can be helpful if a bad cough disrupts sleep. For type A influenza only, two drugs are available—amantadine and rimantidine—that can often shorten the illness, but they are usually reserved for those who, like the elderly and chronically ill, are most at risk of suffering serious complications (see page 30).

## CAN I FLY WITH A COLD?

Unless your trip is unduly stressful, chances are air travel will not make your cold worse. But there are two common problems associated with flying with a cold. One concerns the fact that your immune defenses are already overtaxed and you may be more than usually susceptible to the infectious organisms that can circulate inside airplanes. The second involves avoiding ear complications when the plane descends. When the upper respiratory tract is congested as a result of a cold, the eustachian tubes between the throat and the middle ear cannot equalize the pressure in the middle ear as the plane approaches the ground. The result can be severe ear pain and a seepage of fluid and blood into the middle ear.

If at all possible, do not fly until the congestion caused by your cold is gone. If you must fly with a cold, take an oral decongestant hours before the flight and again at least one hour before the scheduled landing. Also, use a decongestant nasal spray about one hour before landing. *Do not wait to spray until you feel the plane descending.* If necessary, repeat the spray and chew gum during the descent.

To further minimize the risk of ear trouble, do not consume any alcoholic beverages before flying or during the flight. Instead, drink lots of plain liquids, which can help to thin mucous secretions and reduce the risk of a blockage in the eustachian tubes. If all else fails and your ears close up painfully during the descent, block your nostrils with your thumb and forefinger and blow gently until you can hear or feel a click in your ears and a reduction in the built-up pressure.

## CAN I EXERCISE WITH A COLD?

Good news for those addicted to regular exercise routines: there is no evidence that physical activity prolongs the duration or severity of a cold, or that inactivity will cure you faster. In fact, there is some evidence that moderate exercise can boost the immune system and help to relieve nasal and sinus congestion. It makes sense, however, not to overdo exercise when you feel less than par, since excessive exercise can be an immune suppressant and may increase the fatigue that usually accompanies viral infections. It also makes sense to put your activities on hold if you are running a fever, since vigorous exercise will only further raise your body temperature. If you are contemplating exercise while fighting off a cold, listen to your body and do only as much as it seems to tolerate easily. And try to avoid getting chilled. Those who swim should take extra care to keep water out of their nose, eyes, and ears.

## FEED A COLD, STARVE A FEVER, OR IS IT THE OTHER WAY AROUND?

Most people can't remember which way this phrase goes. But either way, it's a myth. When a body is struck by illness, it needs food for energy and protein to help repair the damage, so there are few circumstances where starvation is an appropriate tactic. A high fever will suppress the appetite and dictate a diet that is primarily liquid and very easy to digest.

If the illness involves serious gastrointestinal upset, it may be difficult if not impossible to retain any solid food for a few days. But as soon as this symptom abates, resume eating, starting with small amounts of easily digested foods such as Jell-O, rice, banana, hot cereal cooked in water, and the like. And no matter how upset your system might be, consuming lots of liquids is always very important, and especially so if you are vomiting or have diarrhea.

## HOW DOES SMOKING MAKE IT WORSE?

Anyone with a cold or flu would be wise to avoid smoking as well as the smoke produced by others. The protective hairs that line the respiratory tract are already under siege from the infection, and smoke will further paralyze their task of ridding the tract of microorganisms and other debris. Passive smoking has been shown to worsen respiratory illnesses in children and increase their chances of developing pneumonia.

## Checklist: When to Call the Doctor

While there is nothing to be gained from seeking medical care when all you've got is an uncomplicated common cold or even a run-of-the-mill bout with the flu, there are times when complications threaten that warrant medical attention. The following checklist, adapted from one devised by the National Foundation for Infectious Diseases, can help you decide if a call to your doctor is warranted. The foundation also offers a free brochure "Is It More Than the Common Cold?" available by calling (800) 742-1555.

| Do you have . . . ? | It could mean . . . | Call the doctor? |
| --- | --- | --- |
| Tickly or scratchy throat for less than 1 week | Common cold | Probably not |
| Runny nose for less than 1 week | Common cold | Probably not |
| Sneezing, watery eyes for less than 1 week | Common cold | Probably not |
| Minor headache for less than 1 week | Common cold/virus | Probably not |
| Tiredness, early fatigue for less than 1 week | Common cold/virus | Probably not |
| Sore or inflamed throat | Strep throat | Yes |
| Difficulty or pain on swallowing | Strep throat | Yes |
| Pus in your throat | Strep throat | Yes |
| Swollen glands in the neck | Strep throat | Yes |
| Ear pain (especially in children) | Ear infection | Yes |
| Fever of 100°F or more for more than 2 days | Bacterial infection | Yes |
| Extreme persistent listlessness | Bacterial infection | Yes |
| Severe headache for more than 24 hours | Bacterial infection | Yes |
| Tenderness over the sinuses | Sinusitis | Yes |
| Persistent coughing and/or wheezing | Bronchitis | Yes |

| Fever and/or cough with chest pain | Bronchitis/pneumonia | Yes |
| Shaking chills and high fever | Bronchitis/ pneumonia/bacteremia | Yes |
| Yellow, green, or rust-colored phlegm | Bronchitis/pneumonia | Yes |
| Persistent wheezing and/or breathlessness | Bronchitis/pneumonia | Yes |
| Chest pain that worsens with breathing | Pneumonia | Yes |

**Caution**: Also call the doctor if any of the following symptoms develop: shortness of breath; puslike discharge from the eyes, nose, or ears; coughing up blood; persistent stiff neck; confusion or changes in behavior; or seizures.

# WHAT TO DO WHEN THE
# KIDS GET SICK

I t is natural for parents to want to make their children as comfortable as possible at all times. But when this tendency includes giving medicine to kids with colds, the caring can sometimes backfire by causing side effects that actually make the child sicker. Not infrequently, researchers have found, the main reason children with colds are given medicine is to allow the parents to get a good night's sleep.

## OVER-THE-COUNTER MEDICINES
## DO NOT HELP

In a national survey conducted among the mothers of 8,145 three-year-old children, more than half said they had given their preschoolers an over-the-counter medicine during the previous 30 days and, of those, two-thirds had dosed their child with a cough and cold remedy. However, *there is no evidence that treating children with over-the-counter cold remedies does any good.* It neither reduces symptoms nor shortens the cold.

For example, a study among ninety-six children aged six months to five years, conducted by Dr. Nancy Hutton and her colleagues at the Johns Hopkins Children's Center in Baltimore, Maryland, revealed that those given an antihistamine-decongestant combination medicine recovered no sooner than those who received a look-alike placebo and those who got no treatment at all. More than half the children were better two days after their first visit to the doctor, no matter how their colds were treated. Another study at the Hospital for Sick Children in Toronto found that none of several decongestants tested had a beneficial effect on the colds of preschoolers.

## BAD EFFECTS OF COMMON THERAPIES

Side effects of commonly used cough and cold medicines include fever, hallucinations, seizures, dizziness, hyperactivity, extreme anxiety, tremors, fearfulness, vomiting, lethargy, respiratory depression, and coma. Infants and small children given cough or cold remedies can suffer toxic reactions because their immature organ systems cannot process the medicine properly. Three-fourths of the 76,566 calls made to poison control centers in 1988 with regard to cough and cold medicines involved children under the age of six.

Children should never be given a cough or cold remedy that is sold for adult use only. And dosing guidelines on the package should always be consulted when a medicine is given to a child. Virtually every over-the-counter medicine cautions parents to contact a physician before administering the drug to infants and toddlers. The physician should determine, first, whether the treatment is appropriate and safe for the child and, second, how much and how often it should be given. Yet, according to one survey, more than half of parents had medicated children with colds under the age of five without first consulting their child's doctor.

Parents often misconstrue the benefits of medication. They think, for example, that because a medicine enabled the child to sleep, it had helped to relieve the child's symptoms. But, in fact, many of the cough and cold medicines commonly given to children contain sedative ingredients like antihistamines and alcohol, which in effect drug the child, something no well-meaning parent would consciously do.

## WHEN THE CHILD HAS A FEVER

*Warning:* Do not give aspirin to children with viral infections. Parents still commonly administer aspirin to their feverish youngsters despite widespread publicity about the risk of developing a rare but often fatal disorder called Reye's syndrome when children with viral infections take aspirin. If an analgesic (painkiller) or antipyretic (fever reducer) is needed for a child under the age of twenty-one, acetaminophen (Tylenol being the best known brand) should be used, *not* aspirin.

Keep in mind that fever is a mechanism the body uses to heal itself. Pediatricians say that unless a child's fever exceeds 102°F (which rarely happens with a simple cold) or the child is very uncomfortable, there is little to be gained and possibly something to

lose from giving medication to reduce it. Reducing the child's fever does not produce the improvements in comfort, appetite, or
fluid intake that parents might expect. However, children with a
history of fever-induced seizures should be given an antipyretic.
Give only acetaminophen at the correct dosage for the child's weight
once every four to six hours.

## HOW TO TREAT A CHILD'S COLD

For infants under the age of six months, pediatricians generally do
not recommend giving any cold medicine because of the potential
for bad side effects. To relieve nasal congestion, use a bulb syringe
to clear the nose, administer saline nose drops, and give as much
fluid as the baby will take. A vaporizer in the room may also help to
loosen secretions and soothe irritated tissues.

It is also best not to give anything to older children who are not
acting very ill. If any medication is given it should be used only at
times of greatest need, for example at bedtime or before the child
goes off to school. The recommended dosage for the weight or age
of the child should never be exceeded. Medicines that produce no
apparent improvement should be stopped after one day, and unless
a physician recommends otherwise, all over-the-counter medicine
should be discontinued as soon as the child feels better. Again,
unless told otherwise by a physician, *do not administer over-the-counter
medicines to children for more than three days.*

Avoid combination medicines. Give only the drug needed to
treat the child's most troublesome symptom. Use nose drops for
no more than three days. If an oral decongestant is used, avoid those

that are combined with an antihistamine, but be aware that decongestants are stimulants that can make the child overly excited and possibly interfere with sleep.

As with adults, the best treatment for a child's cold is the application of common sense and practical home remedies (see pp. 54–55). If the child is very tired, has a fever, or feels ill, rest (but not necessarily bedrest) is the best therapy. If possible, preschoolers with colds should be kept home for two or three days when they are most sick and contagious. Give the child lots of fluids but don't be concerned if solid food is refused. Older children with colds who feel well enough should be allowed to go to school unless they have a bad cough, a fever, or some other symptom that would interfere with schoolwork.

It is not necessary to withhold milk from infants and children with colds. It does not increase secretions in the respiratory tract, but it may thicken them somewhat. Counter this effect by increasing the child's intake of plain fluids like water and juice and humidifying the room air with a vaporizer. For school-age children, chicken soup and other hot broths, and herbal tea with lemon and honey, are helpful decongestants.

### Checklist: When to Call the Child's Doctor

Whereas the overwhelming majority of childhood colds cure themselves without complications, there are times when the infection leads to something more serious. The medical magazine *Contemporary Pediatrics* has issued the recommendations that follow.

Call the child's physician immediately—at any time of the day or night—for any of the following:

- A fever in a child of over 104°F.
- A fever in an infant under 2 months of age of over 100.4°F.
- The child is having great difficulty breathing even after you have cleared the nose of mucus.
- The child is so irritable that he or she cannot be comforted.
- The child is very lethargic and can't be awakened.

Call the child's physician during office hours if any of the following problems arise:

- An earache or bad headache.
- Yellow discharge or pus from the eyes.
- A fever lasting more than 4 days.
- Raw, possibly infected skin under the nostrils.
- Noticeable wheezing or a change in the child's normal breathing pattern.

# TABLE 7: COLD REMEDIES FOR CHILDREN

Cold and flu remedies designed for the pediatric set are usually single-ingredient products administered as liquids or drops. Be sure to follow the dosage instructions on the label. In general, the dosage is tailored to children over the age of two. For younger children and for those over two who are very small for their age, consult your physician about the appropriate dosage and desirability of administering the medication at all. As with adults, it is best to avoid using antihistamines to treat cold symptoms.

**Warning:** Never give medicine intended for adult use to children without first consulting a physician.

| Product | Analgesic | Decongestant | Cough Suppressant | Expectorant | Antihistamine |
|---|---|---|---|---|---|
| **ANALGESICS (PAIN AND FEVER REDUCERS)** | | | | | |
| Bayer Children's Aspirin (tablet) | aspirin | | | | |
| Children's Tylenol (chewable tablet) | acetaminophen | | | | |
| St. Joseph Aspirin-Free Infant Drops (liquid) | acetaminophen | | | | |
| Tylenol Infant Drops (liquid) | acetaminophen | | | | |
| **DECONGESTANTS** | | | | | |
| Afrin Pediatric (nose drops) | | oxymetazoline | | | |
| Children's Sudafed (liquid) | | pseudoephedrine | | | |
| Dorcol Children's Decongestant (liquid) | | pseudoephedrine | | | |
| Neo-Synephrine 0.125% (nose drops) | | phenylephrine | | | |
| Otrivin Pediatric (nose drops) | | xylometazoline | | | |
| Pediacare Infants' Decongestant (liquid) | | pseudoephedrine | | | |
| **COUGH MEDICINES** | | | | | |
| Benylin Pediatric (liquid) | | | dextromethorphan | | |

## TABLE 7: COLD REMEDIES FOR CHILDREN (Continued)

| Product | Analgesic | Decongestant | Cough Suppressant | Expectorant | Antihistamine |
|---|---|---|---|---|---|
| Robitussin Pediatric Cough Suppressant (liquid) | | | dextromethorphan | | |
| **COMBINATION PRODUCTS** | | | | | |
| Children's Tylenol Cold Plus Cough (liquid) | acetaminophen | pseudoephedrine | dextromethorphan | | chlorpheniramine |
| Children's Tylenol Multi Symptom (chewable tablet, liquid) | acetaminophen | pseudoephedrine | | | chlorpheniramine |
| Coltab Children's (tablet) | | phenylephrine | | | chlorpheniramine |
| Congespirin for Children (tablet) | acetaminophen | phenylephrine | | | |
| Dorcol Children's Cold Formula (liquid) | | pseudoephedrine | | | chlorpheniramine |
| Dorcol Children's Cough Syrup (liquid) | | pseudoephedrine | dextromethorphan | guaifenesin | |
| Pediacare Cold-Allergy (chewable tablet) | | pseudoephedrine | | | chlorpheniramine |
| Pediacare Cough-Cold (chewable tablet, liquid) | | pseudoephedrine | dextromethorphan | | chlorpheniramine |
| Pediacare NightRest Cough-Cold (liquid) | | pseudoephedrine | dextromethorphan | | chlorpheniramine |
| Robitussin Pediatric Cough & Cold (liquid) | | pseudoephedrine | dextromethorphan | | |
| Triaminic Nite Light (liquid) | | pseudoephedrine | dextromethorphan | | chlorpheniramine |
| Vicks Children's Cough Syrup (liquid) | | | dextromethorphan | guaifenesin | |